高等院校药学类专业双语实验教材

药剂学双语实验

主　编　崔亚男　李万忠

副主编　王慧云　孙珊珊　宋　博

编　者（以姓氏笔画为序）

王保国（济宁医学院）　　　王慧云（济宁医学院）

刘兆明（济宁医学院）　　　孙珊珊（济宁医学院）

李万忠（潍坊医学院）　　　宋　博（潍坊医学院）

张　波（潍坊医学院）　　　张春燕（济宁医学院）

张惠平（济宁医学院）　　　郑增娟（潍坊医学院）

顾英琳（济宁医学院）　　　崔亚男（济宁医学院）

中国健康传媒集团

中国医药科技出版社

内 容 提 要

本教材是"高等院校药学类专业双语实验教材"之一。本套教材由济宁医学院联合潍坊医学院共同编写。为适应医药行业国际化对药学类人才的需求，结合目前大学生英语水平普遍较高的特点，本教材用英语编写。本教材共 16 个药剂学教学实验，包括课前预习、实验部分、实验结论和讨论部分四个部分。

本教材适合高等院校药学类专业使用。

图书在版编目（CIP）数据

药剂学双语实验 / 崔亚男，李万忠主编. —北京：中国医药科技出版社，2019.2
高等院校药学类专业双语实验教材
ISBN 978-7-5214-0730-3

Ⅰ. ①药…　Ⅱ. ①崔…　②李…　Ⅲ. ①药剂学–实验–双语教学–高等学校–教材
Ⅳ. ①R94–33

中国版本图书馆 CIP 数据核字（2019）第 010762 号

美术编辑　陈君杞
版式设计　易维鑫

出版　**中国健康传媒集团** | 中国医药科技出版社
地址　北京市海淀区文慧园北路甲 22 号
邮编　100082
电话　发行：010-62227427　邮购：010-62236938
网址　www.cmstp.com
规格　787×1092mm　$\frac{1}{16}$
印张　5 ½
字数　117 千字
版次　2019 年 2 月第 1 版
印次　2019 年 2 月第 1 次印刷
印刷　三河市双峰印刷装订有限公司
经销　全国各地新华书店
书号　ISBN 978-7-5214-0730-3
定价　**16.00 元**

教材使用说明

本教材适用于药剂学实验单独设课的教学使用。

1. 课前预习　主要是指实验正文中 Part 1 Preview 中的四部分内容。课堂上随堂检查，同时兼顾课堂上的提问情况，当堂给予分数。

2. 实验过程　包括 Part 2 Experimental 中的处方分析、实验具体操作过程流程图的总结叙述；以及 Part 3 中"结果和结论"的描述。也需当堂给予成绩。

3. 实验报告　要求学生在实验课结束后的第二天即上交实验报告。实验报告的要求包括实验目的，实验原理，实验过程（处方分析、实验步骤），实验结果与结论，思考题。鼓励学生用英文进行书写。

4. 关于课程的考核　实验课考核内容包括四部分：①课前预习，占10 分；②实验操作过程及实验结果结论的描述，占 30 分；③实验报告，占 10 分；④期末考核，占 50 分。其中期末考核由两部分内容组成：笔试成绩占 30 分；实验操作成绩占 20 分。即如下所示。

课前预习（10分）

实验过程（30分）

实验报告（10分）

期末考核（50分）　　笔试成绩（30分）

实验操作（20分）

前　言

药剂学是一门应用性较强的学科，其实验教学亦是药学专业的必开课。伴随着世界一体化的进程，以及"中国需要了解世界，世界需要了解中国"的需求，自 20 世纪 90 年代以来，双语教学在我国如火如荼展开。

近年来，在济宁医学院"以研促教"的思想指导下，同时为响应"国家大学生创新训练计划"，培养训练学生自主研发创新能力，鼓励学生积极动脑动手，我们积极转变教学理念，探讨切实有效的教学方法，将药剂学实验单独设课，利用双语进行教学，打破传统实验教学的思维模式，特编写本教材。与传统实验教材相比，本教材具有以下特色。

1. 增设了课前预习模块　①实验中所涉及相关专业术语的英文名称，理论课中已经进行阐释，需要学生在上实验课之前复习巩固，这样可以提高学生在双语实验课中的听课效率和质量。②根据实验内容预设 1～2 个问题，让学生根据理论课所学知识，组织语言尝试用英文进行解答。③让学生尝试写出实验过程中应该注意的关键操作点，然后在听课过程中进行验证补充。本模块的设计有利于教师对学生掌握理论知识的情况进行初步考察，初步评价学生理论知识的掌握情况；同时可初步培养训练学生科研思维的形成。

2. 实验部分　根据药剂学实验的特点，补充了处方分析版块；同时在每一项实验项目下均留出空白处，让学生在听完课后自行画出实验步骤流程图，并标记注意事项。

3. 实验结论和讨论部分　根据实验情况当堂完成实验结果的记录与描述；教师可根据学生的动手操作情况进行当堂评分，可为今后筛选实验技能大赛选手作参考。

感谢各位编者以严谨负责的态度参与本教材的编写工作。本教材各章节任务分工如下：崔亚男（Experiment 1、2、6、10），李万忠（Experiment 15），王慧云（Experiment 3），孙珊珊（Experiment 7），宋博（Experiment 4），张春燕（Experiment 11、13），郑增娟（Experiment 5），顾英琳（Experiment 8），张惠平（Experiment 9），刘兆明（Experiment 12），王保国（Experiment 14），张波（Experiment 16）。

本教材的编写得到了参编院校领导和老师的大力支持，在此表示诚挚的感谢。由于编者水平和编写时间所限，书中不足之处在所难免，敬请广大师生提出宝贵意见，以便再版时修订提高。

编　者
2018 年 11 月

Contents

Experiment 1   Liquid Dosage Forms Ⅰ

——solutions

Simple syrups

Part 1   Preview

<table>
<tr><td colspan="2">1. Key Words. Read the words below and then translate them into Chinese.

solutions-   syrups -
simple syrups-   dissolve -
extractants -   concentrated -
sucrose -   filtration -
viscosity-   sterilize -</td></tr>
<tr><td colspan="2">2. What is a syrup? And what is simple syrup?

</td></tr>
<tr><td colspan="2">3. Please write down how to make simple syrup?

</td></tr>
<tr><td colspan="2">4. After previewing this experiment, please write down some points that we should pay attention to just from your own part of view.

</td></tr>
</table>

Part 2   Experimental

Purposes

1. To master the preparation method of solutions.
2. To be familiar with the function of excipients in solutions.

Introduction

Syrups are widely applied in food and pharmaceutical industry and their consumption is increasing nowadays. Syrups are usually termed as solutions of sucrose and drugs, in which some additives may be included, such as flavoring agents, protectants, and etc. In general, drugs may be extractants from crude traditional Chinese materials, or some others that could dissolve in the concentrated solutions of sucrose.

The preparation of syrups is nothing of special. To be simple, drugs and sucrose could be dissolved in water simultaneously, or drugs could be added into simple syrups which had been prepared in advance. Simple syrups could be prepared just by the dissolution of sucrose in water, in which the concentration of sucrose is destined, that is 85% (g/ml) or 64.7% (g/g). And just because of the concentrated content of sucrose in simple syrups, antiseptic substances could be abridged.

Apparatus & Materials

Sucrose (AR), distilled water, electronic scale, measuring cylinder, stirring rod, electric furnace, beaker, glass funnel, filter paper, cotton.

Contents

[Prescription]		[Analysis]
Sucrose	17 g	( )
Distilled water	add to 20 ml	( )

[Procedures]

17 g of sucrose was accurately obtained using electronic scale, and then was dissolved in 9 ml of distilled water with continuous stirring on electric furnace to be heated. After boiling for a few minutes, the sucrose solution was immediately filtered through a piece of filter paper and cottons which was previously placed and stuffed in a glass funnel. The remaining distilled water was filtered and added to the solution of sucrose. The final simple syrups could be obtained by stirring and mixing completely.

Please write down the preparation flow-process diagram below:

[Key points]

I. The heating step during the preparation of simple syrups is to sterilize the solution, as well as to precipitate some of the macromolecules like proteins. The filtration should be undertaken immediately after boiling. Otherwise, with the cooling of the solution, the filtration will be hardly processed for the high viscosity.

II. In order to prevent the transformation of sucrose into caramel which may change the appearance of the solution into brown or even darker, the boiling time should be monitored strictly.

III. The filtration speed may be varietal depending on the temperature of the surrounding. The filtration could be speeded up by using cotton cushions or multi-layer gauzes.

Part 3   Results and Conclusions

Please describe what you have got in this experiment, and try to explain the problem or phenomenon that you have encountered during the preparation. And please feel free to give us your suggestions on this experiment.

[Results]

[Conclusions]

[Suggestions]

Part 4   Questions

I. Please calculate the concentration of the simple syrups that you had just prepared.

II. What should be noticed in the preparation of simple syrup? What effective steps can be adopted?

Colloidal solutions

Part 1   Preview

1. Key Words. Read the words below and then translate them into Chinese. colloidal solution -　　　　　　　　　　mucilage- homogeneous -　　　　　　　　　　　heterogeneous - affinity -　　　　　　　　　　　　　hydrophobic colloid- hydrophilic colloid-　　　　　　　　　macromolecular – swell-　　　　　　　　　　　　　　thermodynamic stable system- sodium carboxymethylcellulose - coagulation method-　　　　　　　　dispersing method-
2. What are colloidal solutions?
3. Please write down how to prepare colloidal solutions.
4. After previewing this experiment, please write down some points that we should pay attention to just from your own part of view.

Part 2   Experimental

Purposes

1. To master the definition and some of the typical properties of colloidal solutions.

2. To master the types and the typical preparation method of colloidal solutions.

Introduction

A colloidal solution is defined as a homogeneous (such as mucilages) or heterogeneous (such as sols) liquid system, in which the particles are about 1 nm~100 nm. The solvents are almost water except for some nonaqueous solvents. Depending on the affinity of the materials with the solvents, colloidal solutions could be classified into two types, hydrophobic colloid also termed as sols and hydrophilic colloid also named as macromolecular solutions. Macromolecular solutions is thermodynamic stable and the sols is thermodynamic unstable.

The of the two kinds of colloidal solutions is also different. Swelling process is necessary for the preparation of macromolecular solutions, and grinding, stirring or heating is needed when necessary. Coagulation method (both chemical and physical) and dispersing method are usually used in the preparation of sols.

Apparatus & Materials

Sodium carboxymethylcellulose, glycerol, alcohol solution of ethylparaben (50 mg/ml), distilled water, beaker, stirring rod, electronic scale, measuring cylinder.

Contents

[Prescription]		[Analysis]	
Sodium carboxymethylcellulose	0.25 g	(	)
Glycerol	3 ml	(	)
Alcohol solution of ethylparaben	0.1 ml	(	)
Distilled water	add to 10 ml	(	)

[Procedures]

0.25 mg of sodium carboxymethylcellulose was firstly dispersed in 6 ml of distilled water and then the mixture was heated until the sodium carboxymethylcellulose was dissolved completely to form a clear and transparent solution. 3 ml of glycerol and 0.1 ml of ethylparaben solution were then added in sequence. The final mucilage was obtained by adding the remaining distilled water.

Please write down the preparation flow-process diagram below:

[Key points]

I. The dispersion step is suggested to be undertaken in cold water, and then the mixture is heated gently to promote the dissolution.

II. Quaternary ammonium salts and preservatives containing mercury are not suitable in this prescription for precipitation may occur when sodium carboxymethylcellulose encountered with the chemicals mentioned above.

Part 3   Results and Conclusions

Please describe what you have got in this experiment, and try to explain the problem or phenomenon that you have encountered during the preparation. And please feel free to give us your suggestions on this experiment.

[Results]

[Conclusions]

[Suggestions]

Part 4   Questions

I. What is the function of ethylparaben in this formulation? Are there any other adjuvants that could replace it? If yes, give us some examples.

II. During the dispersion process, cold water is needed. Try to explain the reason.

Suspensions

Part 1   Preview

1. Key Words. Read the words below and then translate them into Chinese.

suspensions -   suspending agents -

polydispersity index -   stabilizer -

wetting agent -   dry suspensions-

coagulation method-

flocculating agent or deflocculating agent -

sedimentation rate-

2. What is a suspension? Is it thermodynamic stable?

3. suspensions may be prepared by many methods. Please write down some methods.

4. After previewing this experiment, please write down some points that we should pay attention to just from your own part of view.

Part 2　Experimental

Purposes

1. To master the definition and classical fabrication method of suspensions.

2. To master the quality control of suspensions, especially the calculation of sedimentation coefficient.

Introduction

Suspensions are heterogeneous liquid preparations of insoluble solid particles, the size of which range from 0.5 μm to 10 μm or even larger. The dispersion medium is usually water, and vegetable oils could also be used. Suspensions are thermodynamic instable systems for the high polydispersity index and surface free energy. The main problems on physical stability are particle precipitation, flocculation, crystal growth and so on. To overcome these obstacles during the preparation of suspensions, some other additives like suspending agent, wetting agent, flocculating agent and deflocculating agent are needed. To be special, dry suspensions emerged as an alternative choice.

Suspensions could be obtained by many ways. To be simple, dispersing method, such as grinding and elutriation, and both physical (crystallization) and chemical (reaction) coagulation methods are usually used.

Apparatus & Materials

Mortar and pestle, beaker, graduated cylinder, electronic scale, sulfadiazine, sodium hydroxide, citric acid, sodium citrate, sodium benzoate, sodium saccharin, flavor, distilled water.

Contents

Sulfadiazine mixtures

[Prescription]		[Analysis]	
Sulfadiazine	5 g	(	)
sodium hydroxide	0.8 g	(	)
citric acid	1.5 g	(	)
sodium citrate	3.25 g	(	)
sodium benzoate	0.1 g	(	)
1% sodium saccharin	Q.S	(	)
Flavor	Q.S	(	)
distilled water	add to 50 ml	(	)

[Procedures]

The sulfadiazine mixtures were prepared by micro-crystallization method. 0.8 g of sodium hydroxide was dissolved in 15 ml of freshly prepared cool distilled water. Then 5 g of sulfadiazine was added and dissolved by continuous stirring. The solution (A) was cooled down at room temperature. 1.5 g of citric acid was dissolved in 5 ml of water to form solution B. 3.25 g of sodium citrate, 0.1 g of sodium benzoate, a reasonable amount of sodium saccharin (1%) and flavor were mixed and stirred in about 15 ml of water to form solution C.

Solution A and solution B were added into solution C alternately at a ratio of 3:1 (V/V). Keep on stirring the mixture for a few minutes to form microcrystal of sulfadiazine. Finally, the remaining 15 ml of water was added and sulfadiazine suspension was obtained.

Please write down the preparation flow-process diagram below:

[Key points]

Sulfadiazine is white or off-white crystalline powder, odorless, and will get darkened when exposed to light. It is insoluble in water but will dissolve in sodium hydroxide solution or ammonia. The sodium salt of sulfadiazine will separate out for the absorption of carbon dioxide, as well as color changing will occur for the oxidation by light and metal ion. So in this experiment, the sodium salt of sulfadiazine is not suitable for the preparation of suspensions.

Part 3　Results and Conclusions

Please describe what you have got in this experiment, and try to explain the problem or phenomenon that you have encountered during the preparation. And please feel free to give us your suggestions on this experiment.

[Results]

[Conclusions]

[Suggestions]

Part 4   Questions

I. What are the functions of various constituents in formulation in this experiment?

II. Try to design an experiment to determine the sedimentation rate.

Experiment 2   Liquid Dosage Forms   II
——Emulsions

Part 1   Preview

1. **Key Words. Read the words below and then translate them into Chinese.**
   emulsions-   emulsification-
   emulsifier-   emulsifying agents-
   internal phase-   external/continuous phase-
   oil-in-water emulsions-   primary(Initial) emulsions-
   hydrophil-lipophil balance (HLB) value-
   dry gum method (Continental method)-
   wet gum method (English method)-
   wedgwood/porcelain mortar and pestle-
   creamy white-   Cracking sound-

2. **What is an emulsion? And what is it made of?**

3. **Emulsions may be prepared by many methods. Please write down some methods used in the small-scale improvisational preparation.**

4. **After previewing this experiment, please write down some points that we should pay attention to just from your own part of view.**

Part 2 Experimental

Purposes

1. To master the methods of preparing different type of emulsions.

2. To master the identification method of emulsions based on the physical properties of internal phase and external phase.

Introduction

An emulsion is defined as a dispersion in which the dispersed phase is composed of small droplets of a liquid distributed throughout a vehicle in which it is immiscible. In emulsion terminology, the dispersed phase is the internal phase, and the dispersion medium is the external or continuous phase. Emulsions with an oleaginous internal phase and an aqueous external phase are oil-in-water (*O/W*) emulsions. Conversely, emulsions having an aqueous internal phase and an oleaginous external phase are termed as water-in-oil (*W/O*) emulsions.

The initial step in preparation of an emulsion is selection of the emulsifier. To be useful in a pharmaceutical preparation, the emulsifying agent must be compatible with the other formulative ingredients and must not interfere with the stability or efficacy of the therapeutic agent. Generally, emulsions may be prepared by several methods, depending on the nature of the components and the equipment. On a small scale, as in the laboratory or pharmacy, emulsions may be prepared using a dry Wedgwood or porcelain mortar and pestle, a mechanical blender or mixer, such as a Waring blender or a milkshake mixer, a bench-type homogenizer, or sometimes a simple prescription bottle. On a large scale, large mixing tanks may be used to form the emulsion through the action of a high-speed impeller. As desired, the product may be rendered finer by passage through a colloid mill, in which the particles are sheared between the small gap separating a high-speed rotor and the stator, or by passage through a large homogenizer, in which the liquid is forced under great pressure through a small valve opening.

Apparatus & Materials

Porcelain mortar and pestle, measuring cylinder (25ml), test tube with stopper (20ml), microscope, electronic balance, liquid paraffin, acacia, tragacanth, calcium hydroxide solution, zinc oxide, peanut oil, cresol, sodium hydroxide solution, turpentine, camphor, soft soap, distilled water.

Contents

1. Liquid Paraffin Emulsions

[Prescription]   [Analysis]

Liquid paraffin   6 ml   (   )

Acacia	2 g	(	)
Tragacanth	0.3 g	(	)
2% Methylparaben alcohol solution	0.1 ml	(	)
3% Butylparaben alcohol solution	0.1 ml	(	)
Syrup	3 ml	(	)
60% Vanillin alcohol solution	Q.S.	(	)
Distilled water	ad. 15 ml	(	)

[Procedures]

This preparation could be obtained by the dry gum method or wet gum method.

Dry gum method: This method is also referred to as the 4:2:1 method because for every 4 parts by volume of oil, 2 parts of water and 1 part of gum are added in preparing the primary emulsion. The preparation procedures are showed as below: Mixing the liquid paraffin with the acacia and tragacanth completely, then adding 4 ml of purified water all at once, and the mixture is triturated immediately, rapidly, and continuously until the primary emulsion is creamy white and produces a crackling sound to the movement of the pestle. Then, to this is slowly added with trituration the remainder of the ingredients. Generally, about 3 minutes of mixing is required to produce a primary emulsion. In this method, the acacia or other *O/W* emulsifier is triturated with the oil in a perfectly dry porcelain mortar until thoroughly mixed.

Please write down the preparation flow-process diagram below:

Wet gum method: By this method, the same proportions of oil, water, and gum are used as in the dry gum method, but the order of mixing is different, and the proportion of ingredients may be varied during the preparation of the primary emulsion. Mixing the 4 ml of water with the acacia and tragacanth completely to make a mucilage of the gum. The 6 ml of liquid paraffin is then added slowly in portions, and the mixture is triturated to emulsify the oil. The manipulation is also required to triturate immediately, rapidly, and continuously until the primary emulsion is creamy white and produces a crackling sound to the movement of the pestle. Then, to this is slowly added with trituration the remainder of the ingredients. Generally, this method may spend more time than the dry gum method.

Please write down the preparation flow-process diagram below:

[Key points]

I. A mortar with a rough rather than smooth inner surface must be used to ensure proper grinding action and reduction of the globule size. A glass mortar is too smooth to produce the proper reduction of the internal phase.

II. Before jump to this experiment, the mortar must be "dry", that means in the dry gum method the mortar should not contain water, and in the wet gum method the mortar should not contain oil.

III. Pay attention to the manipulation and the experimental phenomena.

2. Calamine Liniment

[Prescription]		**[Analysis]**
Calamine	0.8 g	( )
Zinc oxide	0.8 g	( )
Olive oil	10 ml	( )
Calcium hydroxide solution	10 ml	( )

[Procedures]

This formulation may be prepared by in situ soap method. Mixing the calamine and zinc oxide with the olive oil completely to make a suspension. Then add calcium hydroxide solution to the suspension, triturate the mixture completely until the emulsion is formed.

Please write down the preparation flow-process diagram below:

[Key points]

I. A mortar and pestle is necessary to this experiment.

II. In this experiment, the free fatty acid is oleic acid and the resultant emulsifying agent is calcium oleate. A difficulty that sometimes arises when preparing this self-emulsifying product is that the amount of free fatty acids in the oil may be insufficient on a 1:1 basis with calcium hydroxide. Typically, to make up for this deficiency a little excess of the olive oil, or even a small amount of oleic acid, is needed to ensure a nice, homogeneous emulsion.

3. Identification of the Emulsion Type

Determination of emulsion type was based on the physical characteristics of external phase and internal phase.

3.1　Dilution method

Add one drop of liquid paraffin emulsions into test tube containing 5 ml of water and shake several times. Record the mixing results. Repeat this procedure using calamine liniment.

3.2　Staining method

Make a smear of liquid paraffin emulsions on a slide and dye with Sudan red solutions and then examine it microscopically. Repeat this procedure with methylene blue solutions. Repeat the above procedure using the lime liniment.

Part 3   Results and Conclusions

Please describe what you have got in this experiment, and try to explain the problem or phenomenon that you have encountered during the preparation. And please feel free to give us your suggestions on this experiment.

[Results]

[Conclusions]

[Suggestions]

Part 4   Questions

I. Generally speaking, an emulsion is considered to be physically unstable, please write down some methods to stabilize an emulsion.

II. What does HLB stand for? How to calculate the HLB value of blended surfactants?

Experiment 3　Preparation of Vc Injections

Part 1　Preview

1. **Key Words. Read the words below and then translate them into Chinese.**

   injections-   sterility-

   sterile preparations-   pyrogen free/nonpyrogenic-

   internal phase-   external/continuous phase-

   thermal instability-   microbes-

   oxidable-   valid clarity-

   osmotic pressure-   ampoules-

   sealing-   check leakage-

2. **What are the chemical characteristics of Vc? Try to write down some factors influencing the rate of the drug's oxidation.**

3. **Please write down the standards of quality control of a given injection.**

4. **After previewing this experiment, please write down some points that we should pay attention to just from your own part of view.**

Part 2   Experimental

Purposes

1. To master the manipulation process of preparing injections.
2. To be familiar with the means to enhance the stability of oxidable drugs.
3. To be familiar with the standards and methods of quality control of the end injections.
4. To master the sealing technique and the usage of clarity testing instrument.

Introduction

Injections are sterile, nonpyrogenic products (or lyophilized products) for parenteral administration. The production material, manufacturing process and quality control of injection must follow rigid aseptic procedures for their particulate administration route, such as intramuscular injection, intravenous injection, and the like. They have a rapid absorption and effect as they are administered into tissue or blood vessel of human body directly, especial for intravenous injection, which are used to rescue seriously ill patients. The requirements for injection are of course different from other solution preparations. The standards for quality control are as follows: sterile, nonpyrogenic, valid clarity, safe for using, atoxic, nonirritant, stable, pH range (usually 4~9), qualified content. And in particular, the osmotic pressure of injection is demanded to close to that of human blood, i.e. isoosomotic.

Vitamin C (Vc, ascorbic acid) is wildly used in clinical treatment. It is recommended for the prevention and treatment of scurvy, facilitating the wound and bone fracture, preventing coronary heart disease and so on. It is reasonably stable in the solid state. In the wet state or solution, it is easily oxidized to dehydroascorbic acid and the latter undergoes further rapid oxidation into the chemical species possessing no vitamin C activity. It is very sensitive to even slight heating, to the light, and to the action of pH and metal ions.

Apparatus & Materials

Beaker, measuring cylinder, scale, ampoules (2ml), instruments for fill and seal, electronic stove, water bath, clarity testing instrument, vitamin C, sodium bicarbonate, sodium metabisulfite, sodium edentate, carbon dioxide, water for injection, steel vase, methylene blue, copper sulfate.

Contents

[Prescription]		[Analysis]	
Vitamin C	5.2 g	(	)
Sodium bicarbonate	2.4 g	(	)
Sodium metabisulfite	0.3 g	(	)

17

Disodium edentate	0.1 g	(	)
Injection water	add to 100 ml	(	)

[Procedures]

Clean the ampoules using swing-wash method.

Weigh Vc and EDTA-2Na according to the prescriptiion. Dissolve the two materials in 80 ml of injection water saturated with carbon dioxide. NaHCO$_3$ is added to the solution carefully and slowly, and with continous stirring. After that NaHSO$_3$ is also added into the mixture. The pH of the mixture is adjusted between 5.8~6.2 with NaOH solution. The remaining injection water also saturated with carbon dioxide is added. The solution is firstly filtered through 0.45 μm microfiltration membrane, and then 0.22 μm membrane.

The filtered liquid is filled into 2 ml ampoules immediately which was pre-fullfilled with carbon dioxide. The volume of the injection solution should be accurate. And be careful of the filling process to avoid spattering the solution on the wall of the ampoule.

After filling out, the ampoule is immediately sealed. The top of the sealed ampoules should be slick, without acrocephaly, bubble or hollow.

At last, the finished ampoules with solutions should be sterilized in circulating steam of 100 ℃ for 15 minutes. At the end of sterilizing, the ampoules are immersed in 1% methylene blue immediately. The blue injections are removed for the sake of leakage.The qualified ones are washed and dried for the next quality checking.

Please write down the preparation flow-process diagram below:

[Quality control]

I. pH value: The pH should be controlled between 5.0 to7.0, comply with the demand of appendix Ⅵ H in Ch. P.

II. Color: The vitamin C injection is diluted accurately to a concentration of 50 mg of vitamin C per ml. The absorbance of the diluent at 420 nm should not be greater than 0.06.

III. Clarity: Comply with the requirements of the regulations of test and clarity of injection promulgated in Ch. P.

IV. Sterility and pyrogens: Both of the two index should meet the requirements of appendix in Ch. P.

V. Other requirements: Comply with the general requirements for injections listed in appendix Ⅰ B of Ch. P.

[Key points]

I. Vitamin C is well known for its reducibility and hence is easily to be oxidized. Such reaction would be accelerated at the presence of metal ions. The reduzates may result in the color change of vitamin C injection. So sodium metabisulfite was added as an antioxidant and sodium edentates act as chelating agents to chelate the metal ions. The metal containers or tools should be abandoned. As an effective supplementation, the displacement of the air in the ampoule by inert gases such as pure nitrogen or carbon dioxide in the process of filling and sealing are also needed. The inert gases should be passed through a washing instrument so as to get rid of the impurity. The sterilization condition should also be controlled for 15 min at 100 °C, which is different from the traditional conditions: 121 °C for 30 min.

II. Vitamin C, also named as ascorbic acid, has strong acidity, which is unsuitable for the injection directly. So in the formulation, sodium bicarbonate is added to convert vitamin C into its sodium salts partly, and the pH could be adjusted to about 6.0 which is optimal for the stability of vitamin C and the irritation during injection could also be reduced accordingly. To be serious, the sodium bicarbonate must be added slowly by complete stirring to prevent inhomogeneous alkalinity of the solution.

Part 3   Results and Conclusions

Please describe what you have got in this experiment, and try to explain the problem or phenomenon that you have encountered during the preparation. And please feel free to give us your suggestions on this experiment.

[Results]

[Conclusions]

[Suggestions]

Part 4　Questions

I. Try to analyze the factors that may influence on the clarity of the injections.

II. Describe the factors affecting the oxidation of a drug. How to prevent them?

III. $NaHCO_3$ is used to adjust the pH of vitamin C injections, what should be noticed? Why?

Experiment 4   Preparation of Glucose Infusion Solution

Part 1 Preview

---

1. **Key Words. Read the words below and then translate them into Chinese.**

infusion solution-   glucose-

powdered activated carbon (pac)-   pyrogen free/nonpyrogenic-

5-hydroxymethylfurfural (5-hmf)-   purified water-

water for injection-   sterile water for injection-

moist heat sterilization-

---

2. **Glucose is easily decomposed at high temperature, please describe the decomposition products of glucose?**

---

3. **What is the sterilization temperature and time of glucose infusion solution?**

---

4. **After previewing this experiment, please write down some points that we should pay attention to just from your own part of view.**

Part 2 Experimental

Purposes

1. To master the key operation in the production process of sterile, and cultivate aseptic consciousness by experiment.

2. To master the manipulation process of preparing glucose infusion solution.

3. To be familiar with the standards and methods of quality control of the infusion solution.

Introduction

Glucose is one of the main sources of heat in the body. It is used to replenish energy and treat hypoglycemia because it can produce up to 4 calories (16.7 kJ) of heat per gram of glucose. When the glucose and insulin are injected with intravenous drip, potassium ions can enter the cell and reduce the concentration of potassium. The rapid intravenous injection of hypertonic glucose injection has tissue dehydration effect and can be used as tissue dehydrating agent. In addition, glucose is the main substance that maintains and regulates osmotic pressure of peritoneal dialysis.

Apparatus & Materials

Electronic balance, beaker (200 ml), sand core filter unit, microporous membrane (0.22 μm), infusion bottle (50 or 100 ml), bottle stoppers, autoclaves sterilizers, pH paper and pH meter, clarity examination detector, ultraviolet spectrophotometer, etc. Anhydrous glucose, hydrochloric acid, activated carbon (powder), water for injection.

Contents

[Prescription]   [Analysis]

Anhydrous glucose	50 g	(	)
Hydrochloric acid (1.0%)	Adjust to pH 4.5	(	)
Powdered activated carbon (PAC)	0.1%	(	)
Water for injection	fill up to 1000 ml	(	)

[Procedures]

1. Preparation of water for injection

This experiment requires a great deal of water for injection. The purified water was prepared with drinking water beforehand. Then the purified water is distilled to obtain the water for injection.

2. Preparation of glucose solution

50% to 60% of the concentrated solution is prepared after the dosage of glucose is added to appropriate amount of the boiling water for injection. The right amount of hydrochloric acid is added and the solution is adjusted to pH=5.0. Meanwhile, activated carbon (1.0 g) is mixed and heat to boiling for about 15 min. Then remove the carbon while hot. The water is added to the total prescription volume. The mixture is filter to clarity repeatedly and the glucose solution is prepared after filling and sealing.

3. Sterilization

Autoclave at 115 ℃ for 30 min.

4. Light inspection

Take out the finished products which with white spots, color points, fibers, glass chips and other foreign bodies.

5. Please write down the preparation flow-process diagram below:

[Quality control of glucose infusion solution]

Appearance and characteristics: This product should be almost colorless transparent liquid.

Clarity: Check the clarity of the product with a clarity detector. The clarity should meet the requirements.

pH: 3.8~5.5.

5-Hydroxymethylfurfural (5-hmf): Take 20 ml of the product above in a 100 ml volumetric flask, add the purified water to the scale and mix evenly. UV spectrophotometry (284 nm) is used to determine the absorbance of the solution and the value should be no more than 0.32 (Disstiled water as the blank control).

Content determination: Take a suitable amount of the above product, the optical rotation is determined according to the described method in Chinese pharmacopoeia (2015 edition II; Appendix VI E, the length of detection tube is 1 dm; Measuring temperature is 20 ℃). The weight of $C_6H_{12}O_6 \cdot H_2O$ is measured after the value is multiplied by 2.0852. The content should be 95.0%~105.0% of the indicated amount.

The percentage of indicated amount = Detected value (g) / indicated amount (g)

[Key points]

I. Pay attention to the quality of raw materials before preparation.

II. Pyrogen pollution should be prevented in the overall preparation process.

III. Filter activated carbon should be quick.

IV. In order to decrease the content of 5-hmf, the sterilization temperature and time should be controlled below 120 ℃ and within 30 min, respectively.

Part 3　Results and Conclusions

Please fill the results and conclusion into the Table 4-1 and try to explain the problem or phenomenon that you have encountered during the preparation. Please feel free to give us your suggestions on this experiment.

[Results]

Table 4-1　Quality test results of 5% glucose injection

Examination items	Results	Standards	Conclusion
Color		It should be colorless liquid	
pH		3.8~5.5	
5-hmf（OD_{284nm})		≤0.32	
Visible impurity inspection		No	
Glucose content		Labeled amount (±5%)	
Discussion			

[Conclusions]

[Suggestions]

Part 4   Questions

I. Analyze the factors that influence on the clarity of the injections.

II. Please write down the standards of quality control of a glucose injection.

Experiment 5   Preparation of Yimucao Gao

Part 1   Preview

1. **Key Words. Read the words below and then translate them into Chinese.**
   Pharmaceutical preparation of traditional Chinese medicine-

   traditional Chinese medicine-   herbal slice-

   Chinese traditional patent medicine-   natural medicine-

   effective ingredients-   effective part-

   extraction-   decoction-

   maceration-   electuary-

2. **What is the definition of extraction? And how many methods do you know about extraction? Try to write them down.**

3. **What is the definition of electuary? And what is it made of?**

4. **After previewing this experiment, please write down some points that we should pay attention to just from your own part of view.**

Part 2   Experimental

Purposes

1. To master the decoction method to prepare electuary.

2. To master the method of measuring sugar content and relative density of YiMuCao Gao.

3. To understand the clinical application of YiMuCao Gao.

Introduction

YiMuCao Gao is the square name, the "red water xuanzhu" roll 20, namely "the ancient and modern medicine complete" volume eighty-five of YiMuCao Gao. YiMuCao Gao as a blood agent, is commonly used in gynecology and applies to irregular menstrual in women. It is made by the processing of the motherwort, and has the effect of activating blood circulation. For blood stasis, it causes abnormal menstruation and postpartum lochiorrhea. The disease sees that the menstruation is less, the blood is not clean and the postpartum haemorrhage time is too long. The postpartum hysterectomy is not all seen in the above syndromes.

It is a thick and semi-fluid leaching preparation made from sugar or refined honey. The electuary is one of the traditional Chinese medicine dosage forms, because of its medicinal properties, it is also known as the oral thick paste. This dosage form is made from concentrated and containing more sugar or honey, so it has high concentration, small volume, good preservation and easy to take. The electuary is suitable for blood circulation, nourishing and anti-aging and chronic diseases. It is usually prepared by the decoction method.

Apparatus & Materials

Electronic balance, electric furnace controlled temperature, casserole with cover, beaker, measuring cylinder, water bath pot, glass rod, asbestos network, 4 layers of gauze, saccharimeter, pyconmeter. Herba Leonuri, brown sugar, tartaric acid.

Contents

1. Preparation of YiMuCao Gao

[Prescription]		[Analysis]		
Herba Leonuri	20 g	(	)	
Brown sugar	20 g	(	)	
Tartaric acid	0.1%~0.3%	(	)	
Distilled water	QS	(	)	

[Procedures]

Soak: 50 g of herba leonuri are put in the beaker, then 70% of water about 10 times than medicinal material are added in them, which can exceed 3~5 cm of the surface of the medicinal materials, and then they are soaked for 0.5 h. Medicinal material can't be soaked in boiling water. Pay attention to add enough water each time when frying.

Decoction: Firstly, the fire is heated to a boil, and then the small fire keeps its boiling water, which can reduce the evaporation of water and facilitate the frying of the active ingredients. After boiling, it is cooked for 0.5 h each time, and then there are twice in all. 30% of the water are used to the second decoction, which is suitable for more than 1~2 cm of the surface of the medicinal materials. Water decoction is filtered with 4 layers of gauze each time and combined. In the last time, when the liquid is filtered out, the residue should be wrapped in 4 layers of gauze, and the remaining liquid in the powder will be combined with all filtrate. The decoction is generally controlled at 1：8 (i.e. 1 g medicinal herbs decoction of 8 g juice). When frying, use water to add sufficient water at one time. Do not add water several times. During frying, stir occasionally to prevent the medicated pan.

Enrichment: The combined filtrate are under 90 ℃ water bath pot, stirring constantly in order to preventing coking until it is condensed into specified relative density (1.21~1.25, 80 ℃) of cream (about 20 ml). The thick paste is dipped in a few drops on the filter paper to inspect with no seepage water mark. As the surface of the liquid is vaporized, a layer of film is formed to reduce the concentration of evaporation and cause the liquid to boil. Therefore, it is necessary to constantly stir to accelerate the evaporation of the liquid.

Refined sugar: 20 g of brown sugar are put in the beaker, then half water (10 ml) and 0.1%~0.3% tartaric acid are added in sugar. They are heated to dissolve until the conversion rate is generally 40% to 50%. The purpose of adding tartaric acid is to convert sugar rapidly into converted sugars under acidic conditions.

Extract: Refining sugar is added in clear cream and continued to refine. At the same time, it is necessary to stir constantly and make bubbles on the surface of the liquid, and so the heating temperature drops with the increase of consistency. Finally, the relative density is in commonly 1.40 or so.

Please write down the preparation flow-process diagram below:

Tasks: In this experiment, you are required to accomplish your tasks by completing the following works:

I. Setting 3 different concentrations of tartaric acid, and try to find out how the concentration of tartaric acid affects the quality of refined sugar.

II. Setting 3 different kinds of heating temperature in extracting under the same concentration of tartaric acid, and try to find out how the heating temperature affect the relative density of the final products.

[Key points]

I. **Decoction vessels:** Generally, sand pot or stainless steel containers are chosen. Don't use metal container or tool such as copper, iron and aluminum. In addition, the size of the container should be appropriate, and the decoction should be covered to prevent the effective components from volatilization and the amount of decoction from decreasing. Before being soaked, the herb is recommended to be properly pulverized (usually No.1 drug screen). It is good for the effective ingredients to dissolve.

II. **Extract the juice:** For the last time, the liquid is filtered out when it's hot. The residue should be wrapped in double layer gauze, and the residual liquid is squeezed out of the powder. Some studies have indicated that the infusion of liquid medicine can increase the 15%~25% of the composition of the drug.

III. **Purpose of sugar refining:** It can prevent the phenomenon of returning sand (the crystallization of sugar after a certain time of storage of the paste), reduce moisture, purify the impurities and kill microbial sterilization. Invert sugar is reductive to prevent oxidation of oxidation. The standard of refined sugar as follows: It is golden yellow and the first droplets of water spread in the water and then round and round. Pay attention to stir constantly to prevent the coking of herba leonuri in the bottom of the pan.

IV. **Experience of receiving paste:** ①When you strike with a stick while it is hot, this phenomenon is "hang a flag in summer and wire in winter"; ②When you dip the electuary with a stick while it is hot and drip on the white paper, there is no trace of water; ③When you put the paste on your index finger and twist it with your thumb and then white silk is pull out about 2 cm.

2. Quality control of YiMuCao Gao

[Appearance and traits]

This product is brown and black thick half fluid, air micro, taste bitter, sweet.

[Determination of sugar content]

The sugar content of the preparation is measured with a sugar meter.

[Determination of relative density]

The relative density of liquid medicine is usually determined by pycnometer method. The relative density of volatile liquid can be measured by Westphal balance.

The pycnometer method is used to measure the relative density of this product: Take a clean, dry and precise weighting bottle and fill with test samples. The filled weighting bottle is placed in 20 ℃ water bath for 10~20 min, inserted into the center of wool stoma cork in order to makes too much fluid from the plug hole overflow and wiped the spilled liquid away with a filter, then the bottle is taken out, dried and precisely weighed. After it minus the bottle weight, the weight of the test can be given. After that, the test samples are poured out and the weight bottle is washed completely. It is filled with fresh boiling cold water and measure the weight of water at the same temperature according to the above method.

Relative density of the test product = weight of the test product/ weight of water

10 g of this product is weighed and diluted with 20 ml distilled water, the relative density should be 1.10~1.12.

[Inspection of insoluble substances]

5 g of the product is taken, added in 200 ml of hot water and stirred to dissolve completely. After it is placed for 3 min, there is no coke and other foreign bodies (trace fine fiber and particles are not in this limit). In addition, the electuary should be checked before adding the powder and the powder can be added after the regulation. After adding powder, the insoluble substance is no longer checked.

Part 3　Results and Conclusions

Please describe what you have got in this experiment, and try to explain the problem or phenomenon that you have encountered during the preparation. And please feel free to give us your suggestions on this experiment.

[Results]

1. Appearance and traits

2. Determination of sugar content

3. Determination of relative density

4. Inspection of insoluble substances

[Conclusions]

[Suggestions]

Part 4　Questions

I. What should be paid attention to in the preparation of the electuary?

II. How is it to prevent the occurrence of "anti-sand" phenomenon during the preparation of the electuary?

III. According to the traditional method, what are the receiving marks?

Experiment 6   Preparation of Acetaminophen Tablets

Part 1   Preview

1. **Key Words. Read the words below and then translate them into Chinese.**

tablets	single-punch press
excipients	granulation
split	evaporability
blank granulation method	deliquescence -
multi-punch rotary press -	screw-
die-	mould-
feed shoe-	funnel-
hardness-	disintegration -

2. **What is an tablet? And what is it usually made of?**

3. **Tablets can be prepared by granulation compression and direct compression. Please write down which is the widest used method, and how to prepare tablets with this method.**

4. **After previewing this experiment, please write down some points that we should pay attention to just from your own part of view.**

Part 2   Experimental

Purposes

1. To be familiar with the basic preparation processes of tablets during the fabrication of acetaminophen tablets.

2. To master the functions of additives in the prescription.

3. To understand the basic structure, working mechanism, and operation method of single-punch press machine.

Introduction

Tablets are defined as solid preparations containing drugs and different kinds of ingredients. The tablets may be round tablets, shaped tablets or tablets with printed patterns and characters. In clinical application, tablets are usually applied in oral, sublingual, chewable, dispersing administration and the like.

The preparation method of tablets may be classified into three types: wet granulation, dry granulation and direct compression. The wet granulation compression method has now been widely used, especially for drugs resistant to wet and heat. The preparation instructions are listed below. Firstly, the drugs and excipients are crushed to the required particle size, and then are mixed uniformly. Much attention should be paid to drugs of small dosage. To attain acceptable uniformity, increment by equal quantity could be adopted. Secondly, the physical and chemical properties of drugs should be considered during preparation, for the thermal decomposition character of some drugs. For some drugs that could easily evaporate may be prepared by blank granulation method. Thirdly, drugs that have bad odor, or are deliquescent or decomposed when exposed to light, can be coated with sugar-film or thin film.

Apparatus & Materials

Electronic balance, single-punch press machine, oven, enamel ware dish, stainless steel sieve, punch, acetaminophen. Sodium carboxymethyl starch, starch, etc.

Contents

1. Preparation compressed acetylsalicylic acid tablets

[Prescription]		[Analysis]
Acetaminophen	20.0 g	( )
Sodium carboxymethyl starch	1.6 g	( )
10% starch solution	QS	( )
To press 40 tablets		

[Procedures]

I. Preparation of 10% starch paste: put about 2 g of starch into 20 ml of distilled water and stir to make sure that the starch dispersed completely. Then the mixture is heated until the starch is gelatinized.

II. 20 mg of acetaminophen and 1.6 g of sodium carboxymethyl starch are screened through a 100 mesh stainless steel sieve add mixed. Increment by equal quantity is needed.

III. The preparation of soft material: 10% starch paste is added into the mixture of acetaminophen and sodium carboxymethyl starch bit by bit. The mixture is kneaded and extruded to make the soft material becomes homogeneous. In general, the soft material should be compacted easily just by a grasp of one's hand and decompacted effortlessly through a mild compression but not turn into powders.

IV. The preparation of granules: The soft materials are compacted and extruded through a 16 mesh stainless steel sieve. The wet granules collected are dried at 60 ℃ for about 1 h. The dry granules are force to pass through 16 mesh stainless steel sieve.

V. Then tablets are obtained by using a single-punch press machine.

Please write down the preparation flow-process diagram below:

2. Determination of hardness and breakage of tablets

2.1 weight variance   Take 20 tablets, weigh them accurately, put down the total weight, calculate the average weight, and then weigh these 20 tablets respectively, also put down the weight of each tablet. Calculate the variance of weight in table 6−1.

Table 6−1   Variance of tablets' weight

Average weight	variance
$G < 0.30$ g	±7.5%
$G \geqq 0.3$ g	±5.0%

2.2 Hardness   Measure the hardness of tablets with hardness tester, usually the hardness should be more than 5 kg and the tensile strength should be 1.5~3.0 MPa.

2.3 Breakage   Measure the breakage of tablets with Roche breakage test machine, the breakage should be smaller than 1%.

[Key points]

I. During the preparation of starch pastes, great attention should be paid to avoid the boiling of the mixture. And during the fabrication of soft materials, the starch pastes should be kept at a constant temperature to avoid coagulation.

II. Be careful of the oven. To make sure that the blower is turned on when the oven is working.

Part 3 Results and Conclusions

Please describe what you have got in this experiment, and try to explain the problem or phenomenon that you have encountered during the preparation. And please feel free to give us your suggestions on this experiment.

[Results]

[Conclusions]

[Suggestions]

Part 4 Questions

What should be considered in the formulation design of drugs which are unstable in wet and heat environment?

Experiment 7　Quality Control of Tablets

Part 1　Preview

1. Key Words. Read the words below and then translate them into Chinese.

weight variation-　　　　　　　　　content uniformity-

breakage-　　　　　　　　　　　　hardness-

friability-　　　　　　　　　　　　thickness-

disintegration-　　　　　　　　　　dissolution-

noyes-Whitney Equation-

2. Please write down some quality standards that compressed tablets must meet.

3. Please describe the dissolution standards in Ch.P. for paracetamol tablets.

4. After previewing this experiment, please write down some points that we should pay attention to just from your own part of view.

Part 2　Experimental

Purposes

1. To master the quality standards that the compressed tablets must meet.

2. To understand the significance of dissolution "Noyes-Whitney" equation and to be familiar with the theory of sink state.

3. To master the basic operation techniques of the quality control of compressed tablets.

Introduction

In addition to the apparent features of tablets, tablets must meet other physical specifications and quality standards. These include criteria for weight, weight variation, content uniformity, thickness, hardness, disintegration, and dissolution. These factors must be controlled during production and verified after the production of each batch to ensure that established product quality standards are met.

The quantity of fill in the die of a tablet press determines the weight of the tablet. The volume of fill is adjusted with he first few tablets to yield the desired weight and content. The CHP contains a test for determination of dosage form uniformity by weight variation for uncoated tablets. The thickness of a tablet is determined by the diameter of the die, the amount of fill permitted to enter the die, the compaction characteristics of the fill material, and the force or pressure applied during compression. It is fairly common for a tablet press to exert as little as 3,000 and as much as 40,000 lb of force in production of tablets. Generally, the greater the pressure applied, the harder the tablets, although the characteristics of the granulation also have a bearing on hardness.

For the medicinal agent in a tablet to become fully available for absorption, the tablet must first disintegrate and discharge the drug to the body fluids for dissolution. Tablet disintegration also is important for tablets containing medicinal gents that are not intended to be absorbed but rather to act locally within the gastrointestinal tract. In these instances, tablet disintegration provides drug particles with an increased surface area for activity within the gastrointestinal tract.

In vitro dissolution testing of solid dosage forms is important for a number of reason:

1. It guides formulation and product development toward product optimization.

2. Manufacturing may be monitored by dissolution testing as a component of the overall quality assurance program.

3. Consistent in vitro dissolution testing ensures bioequivalence from batch to batch.

4. It is requirement for regulatory approval of marketing for products registered with the SFDA and regulatory agencies of other countries.

The goal of in vitro dissolution testing is to provide insofar as is possible a reasonable prediction of or correlation with the product's in vivo bioavailability. The system relates combinations of a drug's solubility and its intestinal permeability as a possible basis for predicting the likelihood of achieving a successful in vivo-in vitro correlation.

Apparatus & Materials

Electronic balance, hand gauge, hardness testers, friabilator, disintegrating test instrument, dissolution test apparatus, ultraviolet spectrophotometry, measuring cylinder (1000 ml, 250 ml, 25 ml), filter membrane, paracetamol tablets, 0.1 mol/L HCl solutions.

Contents

1. Tablet Weight and ChP. Weight Variation Test

The ChP. contains a test for determination of dosage form uniformity by weight variation for uncoated tablets. In the test, 10 tablets are weighed individually and the average weight is calculated. The tablets are assayed and the content of active ingredient in each of the 10 tablets is calculated assuming homogeneous drug distribution.

Please write down the weight of 10 tablets respectively. Then to find out the W_{max}, W_{min} and the average weight of the 10 tablets. To calculate the weight distribution range in percentage terms.

2. Tablet Thickness

To produce tablets of uniform thickness during and between batch productions of the same formulation, care must be exercised to employ the same factors of fill, die, and pressure. The degree of pressure affects not only thickness but also hardness of the tablet. Tablet thickness may be measured by hand gauge during production or by automated equipment.

Please write down the data of the 10 tablets' thickness, and calculate the average.

3. Tablet hardness and Friability

Hardness is perhaps the more important criterion since it can affect disintegration and dissolution. Thus, for tablets of uniform thickness and hardness, it is doubly important to control pressure. Special dedicated hardness testers or multifunctional systems are used to measure the degree of force (in kilograms, pounds, or in arbitrary units) required to break a tablet. A force of about 4 kg is considered the minimum requirement for a satisfactory tablet. Multifunctional automated equipment can determine weight, hardness, thickness, and diameter of the tablet.

A tablet's durability may be determined through the use of a friabilator. This apparatus determines the tablet's friability, or tendency to crumble, by allowing it to roll and fall within the drum. The tablets are weighed before and after a specified number of rotations and any weight loss is determined. Resistance to loss of weight indicates the tablet's ability to withstand abrasion in handling, packaging, and shipment. A maximum weight loss of not more than 1% generally is considered acceptable for most products.

Please calculate the weight loss in percentage forms.

4. Tablet Disintegration

All Ch.P. tablets must pass a test for disintegration, which is conducted in vitro using a testing apparatus. The apparatus consists of a basket and rack assembly containing six open-ended transparent tubes of Ch.P.-specified dimensions, held vertically upon a 10-mesh stainless steel wire screen. During testing, a tablet is placed in each of the six tubes of the basket, and through the use of a mechanical device, the basket is raised and lowered in the immersion fluid at 29 to 32 cycles per minute, the wire screen always below the level of the fluid. For uncoated tablets, water at about 37 °C serves as the immersion fluid unless another fluid is specified in the individual monograph. For these tests, complete disintegration is defined as "that state in which any residue of the unit, except fragments of insoluble coating or capsule shell, remaining on the screen of the test apparatus is a soft mass having no palpably firm core". Tablets must disintegrate within the times set forth in the individual monograph, usually 15 minutes, but varying from about 2 minutes for nitroglycerin tablets to up to 4 hours for buccal tablets. If one or more tablets fail to disintegrate, additional tests prescribed by the Ch.P. must be performed.

How long will it take for the tablets to disintegrate completely?

5. Tablet Dissolution

The USP includes seven apparatus designs for drug release and dissolution testing of immediate-release oral dosage forms, extended-release products, enteric-coated products, and transdermal drug delivery devices. The equipment consists of a variable-speed stirrer motor; a cylindrical stainless steel basket on a stirrer shaft or a paddle as the stirring element; a 1000 ml vessel of glass or other inert transparent material fitted with a cover having a center port for the shaft of the stirrer and three additional ports, two for removal of samples and one for a thermometer; and a water bath to maintain the temperature of the dissolution medium in the vessel.

In each test, a volume of the dissolution medium is placed in the vessel and allowed to come to 37 ℃ ± 0.5 ℃. Then the stirrer is rotated at the speed specified, and at stated intervals, samples of the medium are withdrawn for chemical analysis of the proportion of drug dissolved. The tablet or capsule must meet the stated monograph requirement for rate of dissolution, for example, "not less than 85% of the labeled amount is dissolved in 30 minutes".

Write down the dissolution data of your own tablets, and then determine whether the products' quality is good.

Part 3   Results and Conclusions

Please describe what you have got in this experiment, and try to explain the problem or phenomenon that you have encountered during the preparation. And please feel free to give us your suggestions on this experiment.

[Results]

[Conclusions]

[Suggestions]

Part 4 Questions

I. Please write down the formula that you use in the dissolution test.

II. Try to find out the difference between dissolution degree and drug-releasing degree.

Experiment 8   Preparation of Ointments

Part 1   Preview

---

1. **Key Words. Read the words below and then translate them into Chinese.**

ointments -   hydrophobic base -

water-soluble base -   emulsification method-

semi-solid preparations -   the oleaginous bases-

paraffin -   grinding and mixing-

clockwise agitation-   homogeneous-

substrates-

---

2. **What are ointments? Please write down three types of preparation methods.**

---

3. **During the preparation of ointments, liquid paraffin is usually used as viscosity modulating agent. Interestingly, liquid paraffin is also used in the fabrication of emulsions. Are there any difference between the two "liquid paraffin"?**

---

4. **After previewing this experiment, please write down some points that we should pay attention to just from your own part of view.**

Part 2   Experimental

Purposes

1. To master the preparation of emulsion bases of ointments.

2. To master the analytical method of the function of glycerol monostearate.

3. To understand the definition of HLB value.

Introduction

Ointments are semi-solid preparations containing drugs and suitable additives, namely bases. Bases constitute the greatest portion of a standard ointment and hence contribute significantly to the physical properties, quality, and even pharmacodynamics of such preparations. Different types of ointments could be obtained by disparate substrates. There are three classical methods for the preparation of different bases: water-soluble bases, emulsion bases, and oleaginous bases.

As to the fabrication of ointments, there are three methods: grinding and mixing, melting and mixing, and emulsification. The first method is suitable for the bases that are soft and easy to be mixed with drugs just by grinding. As to the melting method, the additives used in such prescription usually have different melting points and in order to form a homogeneous substrate, the materials need to be melt in advance. The emulsification method is special for the preparation of emulsion bases.

Apparatus & Materials

A pestle and mortar, evaporating dish, ointment slab, water bath, beaker, analytical balance, thermometer, microscope, stearic acid, glycerin, methylparaben, glycerol monostearate, paraffin, vaseline, wool fat, liquid paraffin, triethanolamine, span 80, emulsifier OP, chlorocresol, distilled water, etc.

Contents

1. *O/W* emulsion base

[Prescription]		[Analysis]
Stearic acid	1.7 g	( )
Liquid paraffin	2.5 g	( )
Wool fat	0.2 g	( )
Triethanolamine	0.2 g	( )
Glycerin	0.5 ml	( )
Methylparaben	0.01 g	( )
Distilled water	add up to 10.0 g	( )

[Procedures]

Stearic acid, liquid paraffin, and wool fat are mixed and heated to about 80 ℃ in water bath (oil phase). Triethanolamine, glycerin, and methylparaben are dissolved in 2.5 ml of water, and the solution is also heated to about 80 ℃ (water phase). Then the water phase is slowly added into the oil phase which is kept in the water bath with continuous agitation. The mixture is stirred for a few minutes and is cooled down to about 40 ℃. During this time, the mixture will change from homogeneous liquid to a rough semi-solid state, and at last becomes homogeneous again. The final *O/W* emulsion base is obtained.

Please write down the preparation flow-process diagram below:

2. Fomulation 2

[Prescription]			**[Analysis]**
HLB			
Glycerol monostearate	2.0 g	3.8	( )
Paraffin	2.0 g	4.0	( )
Liquid paraffin	10.0 g	4.0	( )
Vaseline	1.0 g	5.0	( )
Span 80	0.05 g	4.3	( )
Emulsifier OP	0.1 g	15.0	( )
Chlorocresol	0.02 g		
Distilled water	5.0 g		

[Procedures]

Glycerol monostearate, paraffin, liquid paraffin, vaseline, and span 80 are mixed together in an evaporating dish, and are heated to about 80 ℃ in water bath (oil phase). Emulsifier OP and chlorocresol are dissolved in 5 ml of distilled water and are also heated to 80 ℃ (water phase). Then the water phase is slowly added into the oil phase with continuous clockwise agitation. The mixture is kept on stirring in the water bath at the temperature of 80 ℃ until a homogeneous and milky-white emulsion is formed. The mixture is cooled down to room temperature with continuous stirring and the *W/O* emulsion base can be got.

Please write down the preparation flow-process diagram below:

[Key points]

I. The ingredient of the base could be adjusted according to the climate change, that is by altering the quantity of paraffin, liquid paraffin, bee wax, or vegetable oil to modulate the consistency of the ointments.

II. During the process of emulsification, the stirring rate should be controlled neither too fast nor too slow, to avoid insufficient emulsification or inhomogeneous appearance for the sneaks of air.

Part 3   Results and Conclusions

Please describe what you have got in this experiment, and try to explain the problem or phenomenon that you have encountered during the preparation. And please feel free to give us your suggestions on this experiment.

[Results]

[Conclusions]

[Suggestions]

Part 4   Questions

I. Try to design an experiment to identify the type of an emulsion base ointment.

II. Please calculate the HLB value of the emulsifying agents in formulation 2.

Experiment 9 Preparation of Suppositories

Part 1 Preview

1. **Key Words. Read the words below and then translate them into Chinese.**

   suppositories -   nonirritating -

   rectum -   miscible -

   vaginal -   greasy bases -

   replacement price ratio -

2. **What are suppositories?**

3. **Please write down how to prepare suppositories by using fusion method?**

4. **After previewing this experiment, please write down some points that we should pay attention to just from your own part of view.**

Part 2   Experimental

Purposes

1. To be familiar with the characteristics and applications of some popular bases used in suppositories.

2. To master the basic operations in the preparation of suppositories by using fusion method.

3. To master the calculation method of displacement value.

Introduction

Suppositories, which are solid preparations used for cavitary mucosal drug delivery, are usually composed of bases and drug powders or extracts from traditional Chinese materials. Depending on the difference of administration routes, suppositories are usually made into various shape, such as bullet-shape, round-shape, duckbill-shape, etc. The most commonly used are rectal and vaginal suppositories.

Drugs in suppositories should be dispersed completely. At room temperature, the suppositories are supposed to have optimal hardness and tenacity, and no stimulation. When administrated through cavitary mucosa, suppositories are demanded to melt or soften soon, and will dissolve in the secretion to release drugs immediately.

The fabrication method of suppositories could be classified into three types: heat fusion method, cold compression method, and kneading method. The heat fusion method is the most popular in practice and water-soluble matrix or hydrophilic bases are suitable for this method. Aliphatic bases could be applied in all of the three preparation methods. A general fabrication procedure using heat fusion method is listed below: melting bases, adding drugs, filling moulds, cooling, chipping-off the overflow parts, demoulding, quality control, packaging.

The displacement value (DV) is defined as the weight ratio of the drug to the base which possesses the same volume as the drug does. The formula is listed below.

$$DV = \frac{W}{G-(M-W)}$$

Where, W represents the weight of the drug in an suppository; G represents the weight of the suppository in which the drug is replaced by blank base; M represents the weight of the suppository.

Apparatus & Materials

Mold of bullet shape, mold of duckbill shape, evaporating dish, water bath, refrigerator, electric stove, oven, electric balance, glycerol, stearic acid, sodium carbonate, tannic acid, cocoa butter, liquid paraffin, distilled water, etc.

Contents

1. Glycerol suppository

[Prescription]   **[Analysis]**

Glycerol	16 g	( )
Sodium carbonate	0.4 g	( )
Stearic acid	1.6 g	( )
Distilled water	2 ml	( )

To prepare 6 bullet-shaped suppositories in total

[Procedures]

0.4 g of dry sodium carbonate is dissolved in 2 ml of distilled water in an evaporating dish. After adding 16.0 g of glycerol into the mixture, the solution is then heated and mixed with 1.6 g of stearic acid powder with continuous stirring. Stop agitation while the solution becomes pellucid without foaming. The mixture is poured into the bullet-shaped mould and cooled down in a refrigerator. Then the overflowed parts outside the mold are chipped off. The final suppositories could be obtained just by demoulding carefully.

Please write down the preparation flow-process diagram below:

2. Tannic acid suppository

[Prescription]   **[Analysis]**

	Amount per piece	Total amount per 4 pieces	
Tannic acid	0.2 g	0.8 g	( )
Ccoa butter	Q.S	Q.S	( )

[Procedures]

I. Determination the weight of the lank base. 4 g of cocoa butter is added into an evaporation dish and is heated in a water bath. The dish is removed from the bath immediately when the second three parts of the butter have been melted. Keep on stirring until the remaining of the butter has already been melted. The solution is then poured into the bullet-shaped mould. After being cooled down, chipped off and remoulded, the suppositories without tannic acid but only cocoa butter are obtained. Weigh the total weight of the four supporsitories and calculate the average weight, which stands for the weight of blank base (*G*).

II. To calculate the amount of cocoa butter that should be added in this formulation. The displacement value of tannic acid is 1.6.

III. To prepare tannic acid suppositories according to the prescription and the method described in part 1. The amount of cocoa butter added is based on the results calculated in part 2.

Please write down the preparation flow-process diagram below:

[Key points]

I. To make the demoulding process easily and to obtain the suppositories of beautiful appearance, lubricants are needed during the preparation to be applied to the mould before pouring steps. In general, for aliphatic bases, the lubricants are a mixture of soft soap, glycerin and 95% alcohol (1:1:5), while for water-soluble bases or hydrophilic bases, the lubricants are usually liquid paraffin, plant oils or silicon oil.

II. The moulds are suggested to be preheated as high as 80 ℃, and the cooling rate is supposed to be controlled to obtain products of better hardness, elasticity and clarity.

Part 3　Results and Conclusions

Please describe what you have got in this experiment, and try to explain the problem or phenomenon that you have encountered during the preparation. And please feel free to give us your suggestions on this experiment.

[Results]

[Conclusions]

[Suggestions]

Part 4   Questions

I. What is the mechanism of action of glycerol suppository?

II. What is the meaning of displacement value according to the experiment?

III. What are the characteristics of glycerin-gelatin base in suppositories?

Experiment 10   Preparation of Microspheres

Part 1   Preview

1. Key Words. Read the words below and then translate them into Chinese.
microspheres-   pellets-
microcrystalline cellulose-   ethylcellulose-
coated beads-   extrusion spheronization-
centrifugal granulation-
multifunctional microspheres machine-
2. What is the definition of microspheres? And in which preparations does this dosage
form usually use?
3. How many methods do you know to prepare microspheres? Try to write them down.
4. After previewing this experiment, please write down some points that we should pay
attention to just from your own part of view.

Part 2 Experimental

Purposes

1. To master the preparation methods and mechanisms of microspheres.

2. To master the factors that will affect the roundness and the bulk density of microspheres in the extrusion spheronization method.

Introduction

In the systems of coated beads, granules, and microspheres, the drug is distributed onto beads, pellets, granule, or other particulate systems. Using conventional pan coating or air suspension coating, a solution of the drug substance is placed on small inert nonpareil seeds or beads made of sugar and starch or on microcrystalline cellulose spheres. The nonpareil seeds are most often in the range of 425~850 μm, whereas the microcrystalline cellulose spheres range from 170~600 μm. The microcrystalline spheres are more durable during production than sugar-based cores.

If the dose of the drug is large, the starting granules of material may be composed of the drug itself. Some of these granules may remain uncoated to provide immediate drug release. Other granules (about two thirds to three fourths) receive varying coats of a lipid material like beeswax, carnauba wax, glyceryl monostearate, or cetyl alcohol or a cellulosic material like ethylcellulose. Then, granules of different coating thicknesses are blended to achieve a mix having the desired drug-release characteristics. The coating material may be colored to distinguish granules or beads of different coating thicknesses (by depth of color) and to provide distinctiveness to the product. When properly bended, the granules may be placed in capsules or formed into tablets. Various commercial aqueous coating systems use ethylcellulose and plasticizer as the coating material. Aqueous coating systems eliminate the hazards and environmental concerns associated with organic solvent-based systems.

The variation in the thickness of the coats and in the type of coating material used affects the rate at which body fluids penetrate the coating to dissolve the drug. Naturally, the thicker the coat, the more resistant to penetration and the more delayed will be drug release and dissolution. Typically, the coated beads are about 1 mm in diameter. They are combined to have three or four release groups among the more than 100 beads contained in the dosing unit. This provides the different desired rates of sustained or extended release and the targeting of the coated beads to the desired segments of the gastrointestinal tract.

Apparatus & Materials

Multifunctional microspheres machine, electronic balance, stainless steel sieve (20, 40 and

80 mesh), microcrystalline cellulose, berberine, lactose, 25% and 50% alcohol solution.

Contents

[Prescription]		[Analysis]
Berberine	3 g	( )
MCC .	15 g	( )
Lactose .	12 g	( )
25% alcohol solution	QS	( )

[Procedures]

Mix berberine (80 mesh) with MCC and lactose uniformly through a 40 mesh stainless steel sieve, add 25% alcohol solution to prepare soft material. Then deliver the mixture to the extrusion part of the machine to get some column like materials. Transferring these columns to the centrifugal barrel, and microspheres will be got by setting some parameters such as rotation rate, extrusion rate, etc.

Please write down the preparation flow-process diagram below:

Tasks: In this experiment, you are required to accomplish your tasks by completing the following works:

1. Setting 3 different kinds of rotation rate, and try to find out how the rotation rate affect the quality of microspheres.

2. Setting 3 different kinds of rotation time under the same rotation rate, and try to find out how the rotation time affect the quality of the final products.

[Key points]

I. When preparing soft materials, the mixture was recommended to pass through the sieve (usually 20 mesh) several times, in order to make it homogeneous.

II. Pay attention to the dust during centrifugation.

Part 3   Results and Conclusions

Please describe what you have got in this experiment, and try to explain the problem or phenomenon that you have encountered during the preparation. And please feel free to give us your suggestions on this experiment.

[Results]

[Conclusions]

[Suggestions]

Part 4   Questions

I. Will the humidity of the soft materials affect the final products?

II. What is centrifugal granulation method? Try to write something of this method.

Experiment 11   Preparation of Hard Capsules

Part 1   Preview

1. Key Words. Read the words below and then translate them into Chinese. hard capsule- soft capsules - enteric capsules - sustained release capsules- capsule board-
2. What is hard capsule? And what is it made of?
3. Please write down some methods used to prepare hard capsule.
4. After previewing this experiment, please write down some points that we should pay attention to just from your own part of view.

Part 2　Experimental

Purposes

1. To master the preparation process of filling hard capsule by hand.

2. To master the quality control contents and methods of hard capsules.

Introduction

Hard capsules is defined as a kind of solid dosage form in which the drug and pharmaceutic adjuvant is filled into the hollow capsule or seal in the soft capsule. Hard capsules is mainly for oral use.According to the capsule hardness and release characteristics, capsules can be divided into hard capsules and soft capsules, enteric capsules and sustained release capsules. The main material of capsules shell is gelatin, also methyl cellulose, alginate salts, polyvinyl alcohol(PVA), denatured gelatin and other macromolecular compound can be used to prepare hollow capsule, in order to change the solubility or to prepare enteric-coated capsules.

Apparatus & Materials

Porcelain mortar and pestle, measuring cylinder (25 ml), test tube with stopper (20 ml), microscope, electronic balance; liquid paraffin, acacia, tragacanth, calcium hydroxide solution, zinc oxide, peanut oil, cresol, sodium hydroxide solution, turpentine, camphor, soft soap, distilled water.

Contents

1. Prepare granules

[Prescription]　　　　　　　　　　　　　　　　　　　　　　[Analysis]

Diclofenac sodium	7.5 g	(	)
Starch　.	60 g	(	)
Starch paste 10%	moderate amount	(	)

[Procedures]

This preparation could be obtained by wet granulation method.

Wet granulation method: Weigh all the materials with balance.Mix diclofenac sodium and starch well with sieve.Add starch paste into the mixture,and then prepare wet granulation with sieve(18 mesh). Dry the wet granulation with sieve at 60～70 ℃ in the oven. Select dry particles with sieve(16 mesh).

Please write down the preparation flow-process diagram below:

2. Fill capsules

Separate the capsule cap from the capsule body.Insert capsule cap and capsule body into the capsule plate hole,until the capsule body and the plate surface is flat.Spread the particles on the plate surface, gently shaking capsule board, make the particles filled uniform. Put the cap plate and the body plate together, remove the cap capsule plate.

Please write down the preparation flow-process diagram below:

[Key points]

I. Make sure the capsule body and the plate surface is flat.

II. Make sure each capsule is filled uniform.

3. quality control

[surface]: smooth, neat appearance, no adhesion, no deformation and rupture, no smell.

[weight difference check]: (Refer to Chinese Pharmacopoeia 2015). See table 11 – 1.

Table 11 – 1   Variance of capsules' weight

average weight	content limit
<0.3 g	±10%
≥0.3 g	±7.5%

[Checking method]: Take 20 capsule randomly, weigh accurately and record the weight in the table below.Pour out contents (can not lose the capsule shell),clean the inner wall of the capsule body with a small brush or cotton swab, weigh the clean empty capsule accurately and record the weight. Calculate the average weight and compare with each capsule. And there shall be no more than 1 capsule beyond the capsule content limit 1times, no more than 2 capsules beyond the capsule content limit (table 11 – 2).

Table 11 − 2   Results of content limit

Number	Capsule weight	Capsule shell weight	Content weight	Average content weight	Content limit(%)
1					
2					
3					
4					
5					
6					
7					
8					
9					
10					
11					
12					
13					
14					
15					
16					
17					
18					
19					
20					

[Determination of disintegration time]: Disintegration refers to solid preparations should dissolve or disintegrate into small pieces(in addition to insoluble coating material or broken capsule shell)and pass through the screen. According to Ch.P., the disintegration time of capsules is 30 minutes.

Part 3   Results and Conclusions

Please describe what you have got in this experiment, and try to explain the problem or phenomenon that you have encountered during the preparation. And please feel free to give us your suggestions on this experiment.

[Results]
1. surface:

2. weight difference check:

3.disintegration time:

[Conclusions]

[Suggestions]

Part 4　Questions

I. Which medications are not suitable for preparing hard capsule?
II. What are the main characteristics of hard capsules?

Experiment 12　Preparation of Solid Lipid Nanoparticles (SLN)

Part 1　Preview

1. Key Words. Read the words below and then translate them into Chinese. 　nanoparticles-　　　　　　　　　homogenization- 　particle size-　　　　　　　　　controlled release- 　in vitro-　　　　　　　　　　　biodegradable- 　bioavailability-
2. What is the definition of SLN? And try to list some common used methods of SLN.
3. How many methods do you know to prepare SLN? Try to write them down.
4. After previewing this experiment, please write down some points that we should pay attention to just from your own part of view.

60

Part 2　Experimental

Purposes

1. To master the preparation methods and mechanisms of SLN.
2. To master the factors that will affect the particle size in the hot homogenization method.
3. To master the usage of homogenizer machine.

Introduction

Solid lipid nanoparticles (SLN) introduced in 1991 represent an alternative carrier system to tradition colloidal carriers such as emulsions, liposomes and polymeric micro- and nanoparticles. SLN combine advantages of the traditional systems but avoid some of their major disadvantages. SLN are submicron colloidal carriers ranging from 50 to 1000 nm, which are composed of physiological lipid, dispersed in water or in aqueous surfactant solution. SLN offer unique properties such as small size, large surface area, high drug loading and the interaction of phases at the interface and are attractive for their potential to improve performance of pharmaceuticals.

A solid lipid nanoparticle is typically spherical with an average diameter between 10 and 1000 nanometers. Solid lipid nanoparticles possess a solid lipid core matrix that can solubilize lipophilic molecules. The lipid core is stabilized by surfactants (emulsifiers). The term lipid is used here in a broader sense and includes triglycerides (e.g. tristearin), diglycerides (e.g. glycerol beahenate), monoglycerides (e.g. glycerol monostearate), fatty acids (e.g. stearic acid), steroids (e.g. cholesterol), and waxes (e.g. cetyl palmitate). All classes of emulsifiers (with respect to charge and molecular weight) have been used to stabilize the lipid dispersion. It has been found that the combination of emulsifiers might prevent particle agglomeration more efficiently.

The advantages of SLN are: Control and/or target drug release; Excellent biocompatibility; Improve stability of pharmaceuticals; High and enhanced drug content; Easy to scale up and sterilize; Better control over release kinetics of encapsulated compounds; Enhanced bioavailability of entrapped bioactive compounds; Chemical protection of labile incorporated compounds; Much easier to manufacture than biopolymeric nanoparticles; No special solvent required; Conventional emulsion manufacturing methods applicable; Raw materials essential the same as in emulsions; Very high long-term stability; Application versatility; Can be subjected to commercial sterilization procedures. The disadvantages are: Particle growth; Unpredictable gelation tendency; Unexpected dynamics of polymeric transitions.

Apparatus & Materials

Homogenizer, electrical stirrer, beaker, water bath, microscope, Zetamaster instrument, stearic acid, lecithin, poloxamer 188, glycerin.

Contents

[Prescription]		[Analysis]
Stearic acid	2%	( )
Lecithin	1.5%	( )
Poloxamer 188	0.5%	( )
Glycerin (2.25%)	100 ml	( )

[Procedures]

Mix stearic acid (2%, *w/w*) and lecithin (1.5%, *w/w*) in beaker, and then the mixture was heated to about 80 ℃ in water bath until the dispersion bacame nearly clear. Poloxamer 188 (0.5%), the co-emulsifier, was dissolved in 100 ml glycerin solution (2.25%). The melt lipid phase was added into aqueous phase that previously heated to approximately the same temperature. A predispersion was prepared by magnetic stirring and sonication. The premix was passed through a high-pressure homogenizer for five cycles at 5000 psi. The hot dispersion was cooled to 4 ℃ quickly to form solid lipid nanoparticle suspension, and then was stored at 4 ℃ or lyophilized for storage. The particle size was measured by a Zetamaster instrument.

Please write down the preparation flow-process diagram below:

Tasks: In this experiment, you are required to accomplish your tasks by completing the following works:

1. Setting 3 different kinds of pressure, and try to find out how the pressure affect the quality of SLN.

2. Setting 3 different kinds of cooling temperature, and try to find out how the cooling temperature affect the quality of the final products.

[Key points]

I. When measuring the size by Zetamaster instrument, the SLN should be diluted to a suitable concentration, in order to avoid the influence the precision of measurement.

II. The aqueous phase can't be added until the stearic acid and lecithin are melted.

Part 3   Results and Conclusions

Please describe what you have got in this experiment, and try to explain the problem or phenomenon that you have encountered during the preparation. And please feel free to give us your suggestions on this experiment.

[Results]

[Conclusions]

[Suggestions]

Part 4   Questions

I. Why hot homogenization is a good preparation method?
II. What is the storage method of solid lipid nanoparticle?

Experiment 13   Determination of the
Flowability of Powders

Part 1   Preview

---

1. Key Words. Read the words below and then translate them into Chinese.

flowability-

powder -

angle of repose-

flow aid -

compressed limit -

microcrystalline cellulose-

starch-

lactose-

magnesium stearate -

---

2. What are the properties of powder?

---

3. What is the angle of repose?Which methods can be used to measure the angle of repose?

---

4. After previewing this experiment, please write down some points that we should pay attention to just from your own part of view.

Part 2   Experimental

Purposes

1. To be familiar with the methods for determination of the flowability of the powder and the factors affecting the flowability of the powder.

2. To master the ways to improve the flowability of the powder.

Introduction

Powder is composed of numerous solid particles. In the pharmaceutical industry, powder particle size ranges from 1 μm to 10 mm. Powder exhibited different properties because the different shape and size of particles,the friction and cohesion of each particle. Powder properties are divided into two categories:

The first nature of powder (the nature of single particle powders):such as particle shape, size, size distribution, particle density. The second property of the powders (the nature of powder aggregates): such as liquidity, powder filling, bulk density, compressibility etc. According to the flow force, the flow of powder can be divided into gravity flow, oscillatory flow, compressible flow, fluidized flow. Angle of repose and the outflow velocity can reflect the flowability of powder gravity flow, they can be used for the evaluation of outflow capacity from the hopper, motion behavior of materials in rotary mixer.

Angle of repose is the angle formed by the horizontal plane and the powder accumulation layer free slope in the equilibrium state. The commonly used method is the fixed cone method (also called residual cone method). Fill the powder into the center of the disk with a finite diameter, until the powder accumulation layer material along the edge of the disk edge automatically flow out of date, metre the diameter and the height of the cone and calculate the angle of repose.

The velocity of flow is the time required from filling the powder into the hopper to the total outflow the hopper. If the flowability of the powder is very poor and can not flow out, 100 μm glass ball can be added to improve the poor flowability.

The degree of compression can evaluate the vibration feeding, vibrating screen, vibrating filling and vibration flow. It could be tested by the tapping tester. The degree of compression can be calculated as follows:

$$C = \frac{\rho_f - \rho_0}{\rho_f} \times 100\%$$

Where, ρ_f is the close density, ρ_0 is the bulk density.

Apparatus & Materials

Microcrystalline cellulose powder, starch powder, starch granules, lactose, talcum powder, silica, magnesium stearate, hopper, culture dish, ruler, brandreth table, stopwatch, the tapping tester, the device for measuring flow velocity.

Contents

1. To metre the angle of repose of the same material with different shape and size.

[Material]	[the angle of repose]
Starch powder	( )
Starch granules	( )

2. To metre the angle of repose of different materials.

[Material]	[the angle of repose]
Starch powder	( )
Lactose	( )

3.Comparison of different lubricant improving the flowability of the powder.

Weigh the microcrystalline cellulose powder 35 g in 3 copies, which added 1% talcum powder, silica, magnesium stearate respectively, uniform mixing, to determine the angle of repose.

[Material]	[the angle of repose]
MCC+ 1% talcum powder	( )
MCC+ 1% silica	( )
MCC+ 1% magnesium stearate	( )

4.Comparison of flow aid content improving the flowability of the powder.

Weigh 35 g of microcrystalline cellulose powder in 5 copies, which added 0.2%, 1%, 2%, 5%, 10% talcum powder respectively. Uniform mixing, to determine the angle of repose.

[Material]	[the angle of repose]
MCC+ 0.2% talcum powder.	( )
MCC+ 1% talcum powder	( )
MCC+ 2% talcum powder	( )
MCC+ 5% talcum powder	( )
MCC+ 10% talcum powder	( )

[Procedures]

Fill the materials into the center of the disc gently and evenly, make the powder forming cone, when the material from the powder along the edge of the disk edge stop feeding in free fall, to determine the repose angle with protractor (or determine the disk radius and the powder height, calculating the angle of repose).

5. Determination of flow velocity

Fill 35 g microcrystalline cellulose powder and   35 g MCC granules respectively, to determine the flow velocity with the stopwatch.

[Material]   **[time(s)]**

MCC powder   (   )

MCC granules   (   )

[Procedures]

Fill the materials into the triangle funnel gently and evenly, open the bottom outlet, to determine the time with all the powder flow out of the funnel.

[Key points]

Fill the materials into the center of the disc gently and evenly, make the powder forming cone Pay attention to the manipulation and the experimental phenomena.

Part 3   Results and Conclusions

Please describe what you have got in this experiment, and try to explain the problem or phenomenon that you have encountered during the preparation. And please feel free to give us your suggestions on this experiment.

[Conclusions]

[Suggestions]

Part 4   Questions

I. To analyze the influence of the size and shape of particles on the flowability of the powder.

II. To analyze the influence of the type and amount of flow aid agent on the flowability of the powder.

III. What is the main reason of different flowability with different powder?

Experiment 14　Preparation of β-CD
Inclusion Compounds

Part 1　Preview

1. **Key Words. Read the words below and then translate them into Chinese.**

   inclusion compound-　　　　　　　　inclusion complex -

   host molecule-　　　　　　　　　　guest molecule -

   cyclodextrin-　　　　　　　　　　β-CD -

   molecular capsule-　　　　　　　　clathrate-

   saturated water(aqueous) solution method-

   grinding method-　　　　　　　　　freeze-dry method-

   spray-dry method-　　　　　　　　neutralization method-

   heating with seal method –

2. **What is an inclusion compound? And what is it made of?**

3. **Inclusion compounds may be prepared by many methods. Please write down some methods used in the small-scale improvisational preparation.**

4. **Inclusion compounds may be identified by many methods. Please write down some methods used for characterization.**

5. **After previewing this experiment, please write down some points that we should pay attention to just from your own part of view.**

Part 2   Experiment

Purposes

1. To master the saturated water (aqueous) solution method to prepare cyclo-dextrin inclusion compounds.

2. To be familiar with the space sturcture of β-CD and the properties for making inclusion compounds.

3. To master the methods for the identification of inclusion compounds.

Introduction

Inclusion techniques could be defined as an art to entrap one molecule into the cavity space of another molecule. The molecule that is being entrapped is termed as guest molecules, which is usually the active ingredient. To the contrary, the molecules that possess large cavity structures are termed as host molecules.

Many drugs, as the guest molecules, could be made into inclusion compounds, by which the solubility and dissolution rate of the drug could be enhanced significantly. There are also other familiar advantages: increasing the stability of drugs; having liquid drug powdered; enhancing absorption and bioavailability of poorly soluble drugs; reducing irritation and side effects of the drug; covering unpleasant odor or taste; modifying release properties of drugs.

At present, the most commonly used inclusion materials are cyclodextrins, cyclic α-1, 4-linked D-glucose oligomers with a hollow truncated cone. There are three types of cyclodextrins: α, β and γ-cyclodextrins, identified by their different number of D-glucopyranose units. β-CD, which has 7 D-glucopyranose units, is the most frequently used materials for the suitable cavity and low oral toxicity. The solubility of β-CD is the lowest in the three kinds of cyclodextrins which is optimal for the preparation of inclusion compounds. It tends to crystallize from water when the temperature falls.

The CD inclusion compounds could be prepared by different methods, such as saturated water solution method, grinding methods, freeze-dry method, spray-dry method, neutralization method, among which the saturated water solution method is the most frequently used. As to the question of the determination the formation of the inclusion compound, i.e. to identify whether drug is included into the cyclodextrin, many methods could be used, such as microscopic studies, phase-solubility behavior studies, X-ray diffraction, I.R., H-NMR, thermal analysis, TLC, etc.

Apparatus & Materials

Cone flask, graduated cylinder, round bottomed flask, developing chamber, desiccator, thin layer plate, water bath, electric stove, catalytical balance, differential scanning calorimeter. β-CD, peppermint oil, ethanol, 95% ethanol, silica gel G, 1% vanillin sulphuric acid solution, ethyl acetate, petroleum ether.

Contents

[Prescription]		[Analysis]
β-CD	2.0 g	( )
Peppermint	0.5 ml	( )
Distilled water	25 ml	( )

[Procedures]

2.0 g of β-CD is dispersed in 25 ml of distilled water by heat, and is cooled down and kept at about 50 ℃. 0.5 ml of peppermint oil was added drop by drop to the cyclodextrin solution with continuous stirring. The temperature of the mixture is kept at 50 ℃ for 2.5 h. After that the solution is cooled down and kept at 4 ℃ for a night, and white precipitates could obtained. The products obtained are then collected by filtration and are washed for 3 times with 5 ml of alcohol to get rid of the residue oil and dried in desiccator.

Please write down the preparation flow-process diagram below:

[Identification of the inclusion compounds]

Silica gel G thin layer plates are activated at 110 ℃ for 0.5 hour. 0.5 g of the dry products obtained are dissolved in 2 ml of 95% alcohol solution to release the included peppermint oil. The mixture is filtered and the filtrate is collected for the next step (solution A). The controlled solution is prepared by dissolving 2 drops of peppermint oil in 95% of alcohol solution (solution B). The developing agent is the mixture of ethyl acetate and petroleum ether (15:85).

About 10 μl of solution A and solution B respectively is applied on the silica gel G thin layer plate and allow it to dry in air. The plate is then placed into the developing chamber and equilibrated with the vapor of the developer for 5 minutes. After that, the plate is placed into the developer at the bottom of about 5~10mm in depth. Cover the cap and wait until the leading edge ascends a definite distance. Then the plate is remove outside and spray vanillin (1%) immediately. After dried in the air, the colored spots appeared and are observed.

Please write down the preparation flow-process diagram below:

[Key points]

Drugs that are fit for the preparation of inclusion compounds should possess at least one of the following properties: atoms in the drug molecule should be more than 5 and the condensed rings should be less than 5; the molecular weight should between 100 to 400; the solubility of the drug should be less than 10 mg/ml and the melting point should be less than 250 ℃.

Part 3   Results and Conclusions

Please describe what you have got in this experiment, and try to explain the problem or phenomenon that you have encountered during the preparation. And please feel free to give us your suggestions on this experiment.

[Results]

[Conclusions]

[Suggestions]

Part 4   Questions

I. What are the key points in the formation of cyclodextrin inclusion compound? How to operate it?

II. Are there other methods can be used to prepare the inclusion compound? Describe the advantages and disadvantages of these methods.

Experiment 15   Preparation and Solubility of Indolacin Crystals

Part 1   Preview

1. **Key Words. Read the words below and then translate them into Chinese.**

    solubility-   crystalline-

    crystal lattice-   metastable-

    equilibrium solubility-   crystal forms-

    polymorphism-   dissolution rate-

    chloroform-   alcohol-

    microporous membrane-   ethanol-

    phosphate buffer solution-   distilled water-

    indolacin-   standard curve-

    stir-   adsorption-

2. **What is an crystal forms? And what is polymorphic forms ?**

3. **Please write down how to determine the equilibrium solubility?**

4. **After previewing this experiment, please write down some points that we should pay attention to just from your own part of view.**

Part 2   Experimental

Purposes

1. To master the determination of the equilibrium solubility.

2. To be familiar with the preparation method of indolacin's two crystalline forms.

3. To understand the solubility difference of the crystal forms and its effect on drug solution and adsorption.

Introduction

The crystalline forms refers to the molecular arrangement in the crystal substance. In fact, the differences between the crystalline forms are caused by the structure difference in the crystal lattice. In other words, the differences are produced by the different lattice arrangement of the inner molecules. The phenomenon that the same molecule of the same substance can form many crystal forms is called polymorphism. Polymorphism is very common in the solid organic compounds.

Therefore, one drug substance may have different crystal forms, but under the specific temperature and pressure, the most stable crystalline form can be called the stable form and all the other forms are the metastable and unstable forms. Because of the different lattice energy, the different crystal forms of the same drug have different physicochemical characters, such as melting point, solubility, dissolution rate and stability, etc. All these are related to the absorption and bioavailability of drugs.

There are two methods for the measurement of solubility, i.e, the equilibrium and the dynamic methods. The equilibrium method is common in that drug concentration is determined after drug dissolved to equilibrium with stirring the solution under constant temperature.

Apparatus & Materials

Beaker (50, 100 ml), spectrophotometer model 751, piette (1, 2, 5, 10 ml), volumetric flask (25, 500 ml), intelligent dissolution apparatus, analytical balance, microscope (400×) , thermal-stable water bath, centrifugal tubes, injector, microporous filtering membranes, testing tubes. Indolacin, chloroform, alcohol, distilled water, phosphate buffer solution (pH 6.8).

Contents

1. The preparation of indolacin α–and δ–forms

1.1   The preparation of indolacin α–form

Weigh about 0.12 g indolacin, solve it in 50 ml ethanol, the ultrasonic dissolving method was used. Then put it in the petri dish and remove the solvent in the fume hood at room temperature.

1.2　The preparation of indolacin δ–forms

Weigh about 0.15 g indolacin, solve it in 25 ml chloroform at room temperature with ultra-sonication. And transfer to the petri dish to remove the solvent. Indolacin δ-form results.

1.3　Microscopic observation

Put the crystals on the microscope slide, and observe their shapes under microscope (400×).

2. Establishment of the standard curve

Accurately weigh about 12.5 mg indolacin and dissolvc in 500 ml buffer solution (pH 6.8). Transfer 1, 2, 3, 5, 7, 8, and 9 ml of the solution into 25 ml volumetric flasks. Dilute to 25 ml with the buffer solution to get the serial solutions with concentrations of 2.862×10^{-6}, 5.724×10^{-6}, 8.586×10^{-6}, 1.431×10^{-5}, 2.003×10^{-5}, 2.290×10^{-5}, 2.576×10^{-5} mol/L. Measure the absorbance of each solution at wavelength 289 nm in UV spectrometer. Then establish the standard curve.

3. Measurement of the equilibrium solubility

Place the excessive indolacin α-and δ-forms (about 0.3 g) in 900 ml buffer solution in the intelligent dissolution apparatus, and set the stirring speed at 100 r/min respectively. Sample 6 ml solution at the predetermined intervals of 0.5, 1, 1.5, 2, 3, 4, 5, 6, 7, 8 h. Filter solution by the microporous membrane (0.8 μm). Determine the absorbance at wavelength 289 nm using the buffer solution as a control. Calculate the equilibrium concentration according to the standard curve.

4. Data processing

Calculate the concentration of indolacin in each sample solution and fill the data collection table (table 15 – 1).

Table 15 – 1　Determination of different concentrations of indolacin

T（h）	α-(C_0)	δ-(C_0)
0.5		
1		
1.5		
2		
3		
4		
5		
6		
7		
8		

[Key points]

I. The Petri dish should be washed clearly to avoid the influence on the growth of crystalline forms.

II. It is necessary to conduct the experiment in the hood when preparing δ-forms indolacin.

III. It is necessary to use excessive drug in the equilibrium solubility experiment.

IV. Use preservative film to envelop the gap to avoid the loss of the water.

Part 3   Results and Conclusions

Please describe what you have got in this experiment, and try to explain the problem or phenomenon that you have encountered during the preparation. And please feel free to give us your suggestions on this experiment.

[Results]

[Conclusions]

[Suggestions]

Part 4   Questions

I. What are the drugs polymorphism and the significance for study polymorphism?

II. How to measure the equilibrium solubilities of drugs? To outline the precautions in preparing.

Experiment 16   Preparation of Solid Dispersion

Part 1   Preview

---

1. Key Words. Read the words below and then translate them into Chinese.

solid dispersion-   PEG-

PVP-   surfactants-

fast release-   sustained release-

coprecipitate-   melting method-

solvent method-   mechanical method-

---

2. What is solid dispersion?

---

3. Please write down how to prepare solid dispersion.

---

4. After previewing this experiment, please write down some points that we should pay attention to just from your own part of view.

Part 2   Experimental

Purposes

1. To be familiar with the categories of the excipients in solid dispersion, and understand the principles why water-soluble materials can increase the dissolution rate of the drug.

2. To master the preparation process of solid dispersion using coprecipitation method.

3. To understand the characterization methods of solid dispersion, and also the determination method of dissolution rate.

Introduction

Solid dispersion is a kind of solid substance that the active ingredient highly dispersed in the appropriate excipient or matrix. Solid dispersion can be classified into three types according to the dissolution behaviors of drug: fast release, sustained release and enteric soluble release, and also can be classified into four types based on the preparation principles: simple eutectic mixtures, solid solution, amorphous precipitates and glass solution.

The excipient or matrix in solid dispersion can be divided into three types: water soluble material, insoluble material and enteric soluble material. When the drug is highly dispersed in water soluble material, the dissolution rate of the drug can be significantly increased and the bioavailability can be improved. On the other hand, the insoluble and enteric material can be used to prepare the formulations with sustained or controlled release. Furthermore, water soluble materials can be divided into different types, such as: polyethylene glycol (PEG), povidone (PVP), organic acids, surfactants, carbohydrates, polyols and so on.

The preparation methods of solid dispersions mainly include melting method, solvent method and mechanical dispersion method. In melting method, both the drug and excipient are heated together until melting, followed with mixing and rapid solidification in vigorous agitation. Solvent method is also known as coprecipitation method, for which both the drug and excipient are dissolved in suitable organic solvent, and then simultaneous precipitated after removal of the solvent by evaporation, followed with vacuum drying. While in mechanical dispersion method, both the drug and excipient are mixed and grinded under mechanical force for a certain time to improve the dispersion of the drug, and thus solid dispersion is formed.

The prepared solid dispersion should be characterized to determine the dispersion status of the drug in the excipient. The current characterization methods mainly include: differential scanning calorimetry (DSC), X-ray diffraction (XRD), infrared spectroscopy (IR), nuclear magnetic resonance (NMR) and so on. Additionally, the determination of dissolution rate can also be applied to verify the formation of solid dispersions, as the dissolution rate of insoluble drugs can be significantly increased.

Apparatus & Materials

Electronic balance, rotary evaporator, vacuum pump, eggplant-shaped flask, scraper, nylon sieve (60 mesh), mortar, pipette, volumetric flask, beaker, dissolution test instrument, UV spectrophotometer, sulfathiazole (ST), povidone K30 (PVP K30), ethanol, distilled water, hydrochloric acid.

Contents

[Prescription]   [Analysis]

	Prescription 1	Prescription 2	
ST	0.5 g	1.5 g	( )
PVP K30	1.5 g	0.5 g	( )

[Procedures]

1. Preparation of ST-PVP solid dispersion

Prescribed ST and PVP K30 were measured and placed into the eggplant-shaped flask, followed with adding proper ethanol for dissolution. Ethanol is rapidly removed under evaporation at 60 ℃. Solid dispersion could be obtained after the coprecipitates were scraped off and seized through a sieve (60 mesh).

2. Preparation of ST-PVP physical mixture

Prescribed ST and PVP K30 were measured and placed into the mortar, and the physical mixture was obtained after grinding and seized through a sieve (60 mesh).

3. Determination of dissolution rate

3.1　Preparation of dissolution medium

Dilute the concentrated hydrochloric acid 9 ml with distilled water into 1000 ml volumetric flask, and 0.1 mol/L hydrochloric acid solution was obtained (to simulate artificial gastric juice).

3.2　Dissolution test

Measure equivalent 50 mg ST from raw material, solid dispersions and physical mixtures, respectively. The dissolution test was carried out based on Ch.P. 2015 (Part Ⅳ) General 0931: select 500 ml 0.1 mol/L hydrochloric acid as the dissolution medium. The solution was placed into the dissolution cup with the rotational speed at 50 r/min. Withdraw 5 ml solution at 1, 3, 5, 12 and 25 minutes, filter and then accurately extract 1 ml of the successive filtrate to a 10 ml volumetric flask. Dilute with 0.1 mol/L hydrochloric acid to fixed volume for further determination.

3.3　Determination method

The absorbance of the samples (i.e. A_t) was measured using UV spectrophotometry at wave number of 282 nm, based on Ch.P. 2015 (Part Ⅳ) General 0401. After 25 min, the solution in the dissolution cup was transferred to a beaker and heated at 100 ℃ for 2~3 minutes under stirring. The solution was cooled to 37 ℃ again and diluted at the same procedure as previously. The absorbance of the samples (i.e. A_∞) were measured as the 100% dissolution.

4. Notices

4.1　The volume of ethanol should be proper to just dissolve ST and PVP K30, otherwise it is detrimental for rapid crystallization and dispersion of the coprecipitates.

4.2　The liquid should try to keep boiling when evaporation, in order to make the sample loose and the drug dispersed uniformly in the excipient.

4.3　Parallel operation in grinding should be followed in order to compare the dissolution rate of ST, coprecipitates and physical mixture in the same size.

Part 3　Results and Conclusions

Please describe what you have got in this experiment, and try to explain the problems or phenomenon that you have encountered during the preparation. And please feel free to give us your suggestions about this experiment.

[Results]

Fill in the table 16−1 and plot dissolution percent ($A_t / A_\infty \times 100\%$) versus time ($t$), and compare the dissolution rate of each sample.

Table 16−1　The absorbance of ST in different samples at 282nm

Sample ＼ Time(min)	1	3	5	12	25	∞
ST						
ST-PVP (1:3) solid dispersion						
ST-PVP (3:1) solid dispersion						
ST-PVP (1:3) physical mixture						
ST-PVP (3:1) physical mixture						

[Suggestions]

Part 4　Questions

I. How to select proper excipient for the preparation of solid dispersion? In this experiment, why coprecipitation method but not melting method is selected?

II. Reading related books and literatures to further understand the principles why solid dispersions could increase the dissolution rate of insoluble drug. Additionally, learn the Noyes-Whitney dissolution equation by yourself and make clear what factors will have effect on the dissolution of the drug.